Publish

MW00718985

@ Laurence Hunt

Dukan Diet: The Untimate Dukan Diet Recipes for

Lose Weight Fast With the Dukan Diet Plan

All Right RESERVED

ISBN 978-1-990666-58-2

.

TABLE OF CONTENTS

Steamed Mashed Cauliflower

Ingredients:

- 1 log herbed goat cheese

- cracked black pepper to taste

- 1 head cauliflower, cut into florets

Directions:

1. Place cauliflower florets in a large microwave-safe bowl with enough water to just cover the bottom of the bowl.

2. Cover bowl loosely with waxed paper or a paper towel and steam cauliflower in microwave on high until tender, 4 to 5 minutes; drain.

3. Place drained cauliflower in a food processor with goat cheese and puree until completely smooth; season with black pepper.

Jerre's Black Bean And Pork Tenderloin Slow Cooker Chili

Ingredients:

- 3 (15 ounce) cans black beans

- 1 (16 ounce) jar salsa

- ½ cup chicken broth

- 1 teaspoon dried oregano

- 1 teaspoon ground cumin

- 2 teaspoons chili powder

- 1 ½ pounds pork tenderloin, cut into 2 inch strips

- 1 small onion, coarsely chopped

- 1 small red bell pepper, coarsely chopped

Directions:

1. Combine pork tenderloin, onion, red pepper, black beans, salsa, chicken broth, oregano, cumin, and chili powder in a slow cooker. Set to Low and cook for 8 to 10 hours.

2. Break up pieces of cooked pork to thicken the chili before serving.

La Soupe Miraculeuse

Ingredients:

- 1 large cabbage head

- 6 carrots

- 2 green peppers

- 1 bunch celery

- 3 litres water

- 4 garlic cloves

- 6 large onions

- 1 or 2 tins peeled tomatoes

- 3 low fat beef cubes) far too many. too salty... use fewer + taste

- 3 low fat chicken cubes)

Directions:

1. Peel and cut the veggies into equal size pieces.
2. Put them in a soup pot with LOW FAT stock cubes and cover with water.
3. Let them boil for 10 mins, reduce heat and continue cooking until the veggies are tender.
4. This soup is extremely filling and the chunky pieces of the veg are the reason for its weight-loss properties [so don't whizz it up!!]. The liquid and the solid elements go through the digestive tract at varying speeds.
5. The solid pieces remain in the stomach until they are totally digested; they fill you up and produce a physical feeling of being full.
6. The liquid goes through the stomach more quickly and arrives in the small intestine, where its nutritional Ingredients: stimulate the intestinal walls and generate a feeling of satisfaction.

Prosciutto Wrapped Asparagus With Egg

Ingredients:

- Salt and pepper

- 4 eggs

- 1 pound fresh asparagus

- 4 pieces proscuitto, ham, or bacon

Directions:

1. Heat oven to 400 F. Trim the asparagus and season with salt and pepper.

2. Divide the asparagus into four servings. Wrap each with a piece of proscuitto (ham or bacon).

3. Place the wrapped bundles onto baking sheet and bake for 20 minutes.

4. During the last 5 minutes of cooking, cook 4 eggs over easy in a skillet to serve on top.

Oat Bran Porridge

Ingredients:

- Vanilla extract, to taste

- Sweetener, to taste

- 3 tablespoons oat bran

- ½ cup skim milk

Directions:

1. Place oat bran in a small microwaveable bowl and heat on high for 45 seconds.
2. Remove from microwave and add the milk, vanilla extract and sweetener.
3. Let stand for 3 minutes for oat bran to soak up milk.
4. Return bowl to microwave and heat on high for another 45 seconds.

Garlic Oat Bran Gravy /Sauce

Ingredients:

- ¼ tsp. black pepper

- ½ - 2 C chicken stock

- 1-2 cloves garlic -purred

- 1 ½ Tbsp. oat bran -grind into flour

- ½ tsp. salt

Directions:

1. Toast oat flour in 300⬚ oven for 10 minutes stirring every 2 to 3 minutes, let it toast to desired color.
2. The darker it is toasted the nuttier it will taste.
3. Remove flour from oven and let cool. In a 2 qt stock pot add flour, salt, pepper, garlic, and chicken stock.
4. Stir with a whisk to prevent lumps.

5. Put on medium heat and boil until it thickens.

6. Use more or less liquid for thicker or thinner sauce.

Tofu Chips

Ingredients:

- Smoked Tofu 100g

Directions:

1. Slice the smoked tofu as thinly as you possibly can with a sharp knife.
2. The thickness determines a) how many chips you get for 100g and also the end texture (thinner gets crispier and stays crispier) - don't worry about ragged edges as these can be a virtue.
3. quick Directions:s to choose from put 1 layer deep in a hot non-stick pan - no oil required - they'll blister on the heated side - turn after a couple of minutes - do to the level you like put 1 layer deep on some foil under the grill - the upward facing side blisters then you turn - watch like a a hawk! Again 2 minutes each side should be enough - much faster than the

oven, but you can use than too at a lower heat for a baked taste.

4. The grilled version curls up and puffs more and i think stayed a bit crispier -and the burned bits taste like bacon - the great virtue of using a smoked tofu.

5. Sprinkle with paprika or yeast flakes or crushed nori seaweed.

6. If you're counting calories it's less than 100kcal per 100g tofu which makes a good plateful.

7. A great treat for vegans and protein seekers alike - smoked tofu is not the same as marinated - the latter is often much higher in fat.

8. Use a firm version or press it to make it as firm as you can before slicing.

9. Enjoy - would love to hear how you build on this.

Curried Cauliflower Soup

Ingredients:

- 1 teaspoon of ground coriander

- 1 teaspoon of ground cumin

- 2 ½ pints of reduced-salt vegetable stock

- 1 teaspoon of chilli powder

- 2 herb-flavored oat bran galettes to serve

- 1 small roughly chopped cauliflower head

- 2 finely chopped cloves of garlic

- 1 chopped small onion

- 2 teaspoons of curry powder

- 2 teaspoons of grated fresh ginger

- Low fat cooking spray

Directions:

1. Prepare the spice sauce by mixing the garlic, spices, and the ginger and 2 tablespoons of water in a small bowl.
2. Mix well until a paste is formed.
3. Spray the bottom of a tall pan with low fat cooking spray and fry the onions on low heat until they turn translucent.
4. Add curry paste and cook gently for 1 minute. Add the cauliflower, and cover with the vegetable stock.
5. Simmer gently for about 30 minutes until tender.
6. Remove the pan from heat, and blend everything in a hand-blender.
7. Serve solo or combine with proteins from oat bran galette flavored with your favorite herbs.

Salmon Ceviche

Ingredients:

- 4 tbsp scallions, minced

- 2 red chilies, seeded and finely diced

- 2 salmons, frozen

- 4 limes

- 8 tbsp dill

Directions:

1. Cut the salmon into cubes of ½ inch each.
2. Use the juice and zest (from the limes) on the salmons, along with the chilies.
3. Cover using cling wrap, and refrigerate for 3-4 hours.
4. Toss the cubes along with dill and scallions.

Fast Liver

Ingredients:

- 500 grams Chicken liver

- 1 teaspoon Olive Oil

- 1 large Onions

- Salt

- Pepper

Directions:

1. Cut the onion into small slices. Slice the liver into tiny pieces.
2. Warm up the pan at medium heat using the oil. Fry the onions.
3. Half way through, put the liver and dust in salt and pepper.

4. Flip the liver and then cook it to the firmness that you like. This recipe is good for four people.

Ham And Cheese

Ingredients:

- 300 g flour 00, 2 eggs

- 250 g ricotta cheese

- 100 g parmesan cheese

- Half a sachet of instant yeast for savory preparations (8 grams)

- 1 pinch salt peanut oil

Directions:

1. Prepare the dough by placing the flour in a bowl then add the ricotta, grated Parmesan, a pinch of salt, the whole eggs, and the instant yeast for savory preparations and mix vigorously with your hands until the dough is smooth and compact.

2. Let the dough rest for 10 minutes.

3. Take the dough and roll it out on a floured work surface with a rolling pin then, if you have one, pass the dough through the pasta machine until it is very thin.

4. Cut the smoked scamorza into cubes and also the ham if you have bought a single slice.

5. Make mounds of prosciutto and smoked scamorza on top of the pastry and cover with the second pastry.

6. Press down on the piles of filling with your hands and then cut out the stuffed salty chiacchiere with a ravioli wheel or a sharp knife.

7. Create all the salted stuffed chiacchiere in this way.

8. When you have created all the stuffed chiacchiere, heat plenty of peanut oil in a tall, narrow pan and cook the salted chiacchiere

two at a time (so as not to lower the temperature of the oil too much).

9. Fry the stuffed salted chiacchiere for about 10 minutes, turning them with a skimmer, then drain on paper towels and serve hot.

Salmon And Cream Cheese Wrap

Ingredients:

- Cream cheese, low-fat, 1 tbsp

- Greek yogurt, 3 tbsp

- Smoked salmon, few slices

- Eggs, 2

- Chives, sliced, 1 tbsp

- Oat bran, 3 tbsp

- Black pepper

Directions:

1. Take a bowl; add all Ingredients: except chives and whisk well to form batter.

2. Now add chives to mixture.

3. Decant half the batter in a pan coated with oil and cook until both sides are golden.
4. Do the same for remaining batter.
5. Arrange pancakes in a serving dish and keep aside to cool for few minutes.
6. Press with cream and add salmon topping.
7. Season with pepper before you fold and serve.

Chicken Rillettes

Ingredients:

- 5 gherkin pickles*

- ½ cup fat-free plain Greek-style yogurt

- A pinch of chili powder

- A pinch of ground or grated nutmeg

- ⅛ teaspoon vegetable oil

- 1 pound boneless, skinless chicken or turkey breast, cut into ½-inch cubes

- 2 onions, roughly chopped

- Salt and freshly ground black pepper

Directions:

1. Heat a heavy-bottomed frying pan over high heat.
2. Add the oil and wipe out any excess with a paper towel.
3. Add the chicken pieces and cook, stirring often, for 5 minutes, or until brown.
4. Place the chicken pieces, onions, gherkins, yogurt, chili powder, and nutmeg in a food processor and blend, pulsing on and off, until the texture is smooth, but still thick and somewhat textured.
5. Add salt and pepper to taste.
6. Place the chicken mixture into a loaf pan, packing it tightly.
7. Cover and refrigerate for at least 2 hours before serving.

Chicken Tacos

Ingredients:

- Chopped onions

- Dried chili pepper

- Garlic powder

- 1teaspoon baking powder

- 2 tablespoons of oat bran and 1 of wheat bran

- 1 egg

- 2 tablespoons of 0 fat greek yogurt

Directions:

1. Spray of some spray oil – or a couple of drops of oil in the pan then mopped with kitchen towel

2. Heated up the pan and spooned in 1/2 the mix and spread it aroud really thin. Made 2 soft tacos

Easy Grillin' Burgers

Ingredients:

- Ground 1 clove garlic, finely

- Cleaved 2 eggs, beaten

- Sea salt and newly ground dark pepper

- 2lbs ground beef

- 1 enormous onion, coarsely

Directions:

1. Put hamburger in a huge bowl along with the coarsely ground onion and finely hacked garlic, Add salt and pepper.
2. Join eggs until well distributed. Mold burgers by taking a small bunch of the hamburger blend and folding it into a ball.

3. Straighten the ball on a plate or level work area.

4. Preferably, the burger will be around 1 inch thick.

Simple Fruit Dip

Ingredients:

- ⅓ cup packed brown sugar

- 1 teaspoon caramelized sugar

- 8 ounces cream cheese

- 2 tablespoons white sugar

Directions:

1. Combine the cream cheese, white sugar, brown sugar and caramelized sugar. Beat until smooth.
2. Serve with fresh fruit for dipping.

Creamy Vanilla Fruit Dip

Ingredients:

- 1 teaspoon vanilla extract

- 1 (12 ounce) container frozen whipped topping, thawed

- 1 (8 ounce) package cream cheese, softened

- ½ cup confectioners' sugar

Directions:

1. Cream together the cream cheese and sugar until well combined.
2. Stir in the vanilla extract and then the whipped topping. Chill in refrigerator 1 hour.

Grilled "Tandoori" Lamb

Ingredients:

- ½ teaspoon cayenne pepper

- 2 pounds boneless lamb shoulder, cut into 2 inch pieces

- 2 teaspoons kosher salt, divided

- 1 tablespoon vegetable oil

- ½ cup chopped cilantro

- 4 small fresh lemon wedges

- 1 medium red onion, sliced

- spicy cilantro chutney

- 1 cup plain yogurt

- ½ cup lemon juice

- ¼ cup finely minced onion

- 2 cloves crushed garlic

- 1 tablespoon freshly grated ginger

- 2 teaspoons garam masala

- 2 teaspoons paprika

- 1 teaspoon ground cumin

- ½ teaspoon turmeric powder

Directions:

1. Whisk yogurt, lemon juice, onion, garlic, ginger, garam masala, paprika, cumin, turmeric, and cayenne pepper together in a bowl until combined.
2. Toss lamb and salt into marinade; mix until lamb pieces are coated evenly.
3. Cover mixture with plastic wrap and refrigerate overnight, or at least 4 hours.

31

4. Skewer lamb pieces so they barely touch. Wipe off excess marinade with a paper towel. Brush with vegetable oil and sprinkle with salt.
5. Preheat grill for medium heat and lightly oil the grate.
6. Grill skewers on medium heat until lamb springs back to the touch, about 5 to 7 minutes on each side.
7. Garnish with red onions, lemon wedges, and chopped cilantro as desired .

Creamy Chicken And Broccoli Curry

Ingredients:

- 1 1/2 cups broccoli, steamed

- 1/2 cup fat-free sour cream

- 1 t cornstarch, mixed in 1/4 cup water

- Olive oil spray

- Salt and pepper

- 1 1/2 lbs chicken tenders

- 1 onion, chopped

- 1 1/2 t curry powder, any that you like

- 1 1/2 cups chicken broth

Directions:

1. Season tenders with salt and pepper, a bit of olive oil spray and brown in a skillet for 3 minutes per side. Transfer chicken to a plate.
2. Add onion to the skillet and a bit of olive oil spray and cook for five minutes.
3. Add broth, cornstarch slurry, curry powder and season with salt and pepper.
4. Cook for another 3-5 minutes or until the sauce has thickened a bit.
5. Return the chicken to the skillet, add the broccoli and heat for 2-3 minutes.
6. Remove from heat and stir in the sour cream.

Dukan Beef Kebabs

Ingredients:

For the marinade:

- ½ teaspoon ginger

- 1 pinch of cayenne pepper

- salt

- 1 teaspoon sweetener

- 3 tablespoon low sodium soy sauce (sugar free)

- 3 tablespoon lemon juice

- 2 garlic cloves, finely chopped

For the kebabs:

- 1 onion cut into large chunks

- 1 bell pepper (green, red or yellow), seeds removed and cut into large chunks

- 6 wooden kebab skewers

- 300 g lean beef (top sirloin or tenderloin), cut into large cubes

- 2 tomatoes cut into large chunks

Directions:

1. In a large mixing bowl, mix together all the Ingredients: for the marinade.
2. Transfer the cubed beef into the mixture, stir to coat and let it marinate for 3 hours, giving it a stir every hour.
3. Preheat the oven to 350 F/180 C.
4. Thread the beef cubes and vegetables onto the kebab sticks in an alternating order.
5. Place them in a non-stick oven proof dish and cook for 20 minutes, turning frequently to ensure all sides are cooked evenly.

Diet Mayonnaise

Ingredients:

- Salt and freshly ground black pepper, to taste

- 3 tablespoons zero fat Greek yogurt

- 1 egg yolk

- 1 tablespoon Dijon mustard

Directions:

1. Put egg yolk in small bowl and beat gently.
2. Add Dijon mustard, salt and pepper and any other seasoning of your choice and mix well.
3. Add the Greek yogurt a little bit at a time, stirring constantly, until all the Ingredients: are well-combined.
4. Refrigerate in an airtight container.

Lemon Oat Bran Gravy /Sauce

Ingredients:

- ¼ tsp. black pepper

- ½ tsp. lemon zest

- 2 Tbsp. fresh lemon juice

- 1 ½ Tbsp. oat bran -grind into flour

- ½ - 2 chicken or vegetable stock

- ½ tsp. salt

Directions:

1. Toast oat flour in 300⬚ oven for 10 minutes stirring every 2 to 3 minutes, let it toast to desired color.

2. The darker it is toasted the nuttier it will taste.

3. Remove flour from oven and let cool. In a 2 qt stock pot add flour, salt, pepper, lemon zest,

lemon juice, and chicken stock. Stir with a whisk to prevent lumps.

4. Put on medium heat and boil until it thickens.
5. Use more or less liquid for thicker or thinner sauce.

Choco-Raspberry And Choco-Mint Cupcakes

Ingredients:

- 2 tbsp fat-free fromage frais

- 4 eggs

- 10 tsp Canderel granules

- 6 drops red-pink food colouring

- ½ tsp raspberry flavouring

- 6 drops green food colouring

- ½ tsp peppermint flavouring

- 4 tbsp powdered skimmed milk

- 4 tbsp oat bran

- 2 tbsp wheat bran

- 4 tsp sugar-free reduced-fat cocoa powder

- 2 tsp liquid Hermesetas

- 1 × 8g sachet baking powder

Directions:

1. Preheat the oven to 180C/Gas 4. In a bowl, stir together the oat and wheat brans, cocoa powder and liquid sweetener.

2. Next add the baking powder and fromage frais. Break 2 of the eggs into a bowl, separating the whites from the yolks.

3. Put the whites to one side. Add yolks to the bran mixture along with the remaining 2 whole eggs.

4. Pour the bran mixture into silicone muffin moulds and bake in the preheated oven for 15 minutes, keeping a careful eye on the cupcakes to check when they are ready.

5. In the meantime, make the icing. Add the Canderel granules to the reserved egg whites.

6. Divide the egg whites between two bowls.

7. To one bowl, add the red-pink food colouring and the raspberry flavouring and to the other bowl, add the green food colouring and the peppermint flavouring.

8. Finely blend the powdered milk and sprinkle carefully into both bowls, stirring gradually until you get the nice thick texture of traditional icing.

9. Ice half the cupcakes with the raspberry icing and the other half with the peppermint icing.

10. Put the cupcakes in the fridge to allow the icing to harden and decorate with fruit and peppermint leaves.

Sage And Butternut Squash Soup

Ingredients:

- ½ onion, chopped

- Freshly ground black pepper

- Low fat cooking spray

- 2 herb-flavored oat bran galettes to serve (optional)

- A handful of fresh sage leaves

- 2 small peeled, de-seeded butternut squashes cut into large chunks

- 2 ½ pints of reduced salt chicken stock

Directions:

1. Pre-heat the oven to 200 degrees Celsius. Line a baking tray with greaseproof paper.

2. Put the butternut squash in a tray, spread the sage leaves uniformly over the squash, add some freshly ground black pepper and spray with low fat cooking spray.

3. Slide the tray into the oven to cook for about 40 minutes, or until the sage leaves are crispy and the butternut squash turns tender.

4. Before the squash is set, find a tall pan and spray the bottom with low fat cooking spray, and fry the onions under medium heat until translucent.

5. Transfer the sage leaves and the butternut squash into the pan and cover.

6. Simmer for 15 minutes. Remove the pan from heat then put its contents in a blender and blend until smooth.

7. Serve on its own or flavor with oat bran galette flavored with your favorite herbs.

Garlic And Dill Chicken Breasts

Ingredients:

- 1 tbsp fresh dill, chopped

- 1 onion, finely diced

- 1 tsp rapeseed oil

- ½ tbsp lemon juice

- 1 tsp corn flour

- 2 chicken breasts, skinless and boneless

- ½ cup chicken stock

- 2 cloves of garlic, minced

- Salt, to taste

- Pepper, to taste

Directions:

1. Cook the chicken breast in a pan, for about 3-4 minutes on each side – till it becomes brown.
2. In another pan, add some oil and then cook garlic and onion for 3-4 more minutes.
3. In a bowl, mix the chicken stock, dill, lemon juice and corn flour.
4. Add this to the pan with the onion and stir till the corn flour mix becomes thick – add salt and pepper according to taste.
5. Add the chicken to this pan, and let it cook some more – for about 5 minutes.
6. Garnish with some more fresh dill.

Fiber Bread

Ingredients:

- A pinch of Ginger and linseed

- 2 spoons of nonfat Natural yoghurt

- 16 spoons of Oat bran

- 8 spoons Wheat Bran

- A pinch of Cayenne pepper

- 250 grams nonfat Cottage Cheese

- A pinch of Cumin and salt

- 6 Eggs

Directions:

1. Toss well all the Ingredients: and put into a short fruitcake-form with cooking paper.

2. Dust the top with linseed. You can use goji berries, pumpkin seeds or sunflower seeds into the bread.
3. Cook in the oven for 20 minutes at 220◦C then lessen temperature to 180◦C and cook for another 20 minutes.
4. Turn off the cooker without taking the bread from the oven for another 20 minutes.

Madame Croque

Ingredients:

- 100 g Gruyère

- 4 eggs 50 g butter

- 8 slices of toast

- 4 slices cooked ham

Directions:

Prepare the toast

1. Take half of the butter and melt it completely. Place half of the toast slices on a baking sheet with baking paper and brush them with melted butter and brown them in the oven for 5 minutes.

2. Place the ham slices on top of the butter brushed slices.

3. Grate the Gruyere cheese with a wide-hole grater and spread it evenly over the cooked ham.
4. Take the remaining slices of bacon and place them on top to create a toast.

Prepare the fried egg

1. In a non-stick pan, melt the remaining amount of butter.
2. Remove the fried egg from the frying pan and place it on a plate.in the same frying pan where you cooked the egg and where a little melted butter remains, brown the toast on both sides, then remove from the pan and place on a plate.
3. Place the fried egg on top of each piece of toast and serve the Croque madame piping hot.

Oat Bran Galette With Toffee Yogurt

Ingredients:

- Toffee yogurt, low-fat, 1 small pot

- Greek yogurt, 2 tbsp

- Sweetener, 1 tsp

- Egg, 1

- Oat bran, 2 tbsp

Directions:

1. Take a bowl; add egg, oat bran, sweetener as well as yogurt and combine.
2. Add half the mixture in a frying pan coated with oil and cook pancakes on medium high heat until golden.
3. Arrange onto platters; wrap it with lid and do the same with remaining mixture.
4. Serve alongside toffee yogurt.

Sautéed Chicken With Lemon And Capers

Ingredients:

- Grated zest of 1 lemon

- 1 tablespoon small capers, drained and rinsed

- 1 tablespoon fresh lemon juice

- 5 fresh basil leaves, finely chopped

- ⅛ teaspoon vegetable oil

- 1 small red onion, finely chopped

- 1 pound½ boneless, skinless chicken breasts, cut into thin slices across the grain of the meat

- Salt and freshly ground black pepper

Directions:

1. Heat a nonstick, heavy-bottomed frying pan over medium heat. Add the oil and wipe out any excess with a paper towel.

2. Add the onion and cook, stirring often, until it turns golden brown. Remove from the pan and reserve.

3. Add the chicken slices to the same pan and cook, stirring often, until browned, about 7 minutes.

4. Add the reserved onion, lemon zest, capers, lemon juice, and basil, and stir thoroughly. Add salt and pepper to taste.

Chicken Kiev

Ingredients:

- Salt and pepper,

- 1 egg

- 2 slices DD bread, crumbed,

- Spray light or similar

- Chicken breast ,

- Extra low fat laughing cow,

- 1/4 teaspoon dried parsley

- 1/4 teaspoon garlic granules,

Directions:

1. Slice into the chicken breast at the thickest point to make a little pocket, mash the laughing cow cheese with the parsley and

garlic until well blended, put it into the 'pocket' close it up with 2 wooden cocktail sticks or tie it with string.

2. Beat the egg, then dip the chicken into it, then dip the chicken into the breadcrumbs, pressing them down lightly all over the chicken, lightly spray the baking tray, put the chicken onto the baking tray cocktail stick side up, lightly spray the chicken with frylight , Bake for 30-35mins at 200C. delicious hot or cold

Savory Ginger-Beef Stir-Fry

Ingredients:

- ¼ c. clam sauce

- 1" shape of ginger, finely slashed 2 garlic cloves, crushed

- Freshly ground dark pepper

- 414oz meat filet, cut into slight strips 1 huge onion, finely

- Chopped

- ¼ c. soy sauce

Directions:

1. Assemble marinade by consolidating soy sauce, shellfish sauce, ginger, pepper and garlic together in a bowl.
2. Add the cuts of hamburger and refrigerate for 60 minutes.
3. Dry fry onions in a skillet until delicate and.
4. Then, at that point, add hamburger strips to onions and cook until there is no noticeable pink.

Tuna Casserole With Shirataki Noodles

Ingredients:

- 1 (8 ounce) package shirataki noodles (such as Miracle Noodles®)

- ½ cup almond milk (such as Silk®)

- 2 tablespoons light vegetable cream cheese

- 1 teaspoon seafood seasoning (such as Old Bay®)

- ½ teaspoon garlic powder

- ⅛ teaspoon ground black pepper

- 1 (7 ounce) can yellowfin tuna, drained

- ½ (12 ounce) package fresh green beans, trimmed

- ¾ cup sliced red bell pepper

- ⅓ cup chopped onion

- ½ cup sliced fresh mushrooms

Directions:

1. Place green beans in a large pot and cover with salted water; bring to a boil.
2. Reduce heat to medium-low and simmer until tender yet firm to the bite, about 5 minutes. Drain.
3. Cook and stir red bell pepper and onion in a large nonstick skillet until tender, about 5 minutes.
4. Add mushrooms; cook for 3 to 4 minutes.
5. While mushrooms are cooking, drain and rinse noodles; set aside.
6. Combine almond milk, cream cheese, seafood seasoning, garlic powder, and pepper in a blender; blend until smooth.
7. Add greens beans, noodles, cream cheese mixture, and tuna to the mushroom mixture.

8. Stir gently until heated through, 5 to 8 minutes.

Fruity Curry Chicken Salad

Ingredients:

- ⅓ cup golden raisins

- ⅓ cup seedless green grapes, halved

- ½ cup chopped toasted pecans

- ⅛ teaspoon ground black pepper

- ½ teaspoon curry powder

- 4 skinless, boneless chicken breast halves - cooked and diced

- 1 stalk celery, diced

- 4 green onions, chopped

- 1 Golden Delicious apple - peeled, cored and diced

- ¾ cup light mayonnaise

Directions:

1. In a large bowl combine the chicken, celery, onion, apple, raisins, grapes, pecans, pepper, curry powder and mayonnaise. Mix all together. Serve!

Cinnamon Sugar Flatbread

Ingredients:

- 1/2 t olive oil

- 2 t splenda, divded

- 1 t cinnamon

- Pinch of freshly ground nutmeg

- 1 packet of rapid rise active yeast

- 1/4 cup warm water

- 1/4 cup of oat bran, ground in a coffee grinder to flour consistency

- A pinch of salt

Directions:

1. Activate the yeast in the warm water and whisk until disolved. In a double boiler over

simmering water, add yeast to the flour, salt, 1 teaspoon of Splenda, a 1/4 teaspoon of cinnamon and olive oil, slowly, until a very sticky ball of dough forms.

2. Spray a glass bowl with olive oil spray, place the dough in the bowl, cover with a kitchen towel and let rise in a warm place for an hour.

3. The dough will not rise much but it will lose it's stickiness and become much easier to handle.

4. Sprinkle some oat bran on a cutting board and roll out the dough until it's cracker-thin (should be about a 7-inch circle).

5. Cut the dough into 2-inch wide strips.

6. Spray with olive oil spray and sprinkle with Splenda, cinnamon and nutmeg.

7. Place on a pizza stone or cookie sheet and bake at 425 for twelve minutes. Eat hot out of the oven.

Dukan Lasagna

Ingredients:

For filling:

- 10 ounces tomato sauce

- 5 ounces tomato paste

- ½ cup water

- salt, pepper, dry basil

- 3 tbsp chopped fresh parsley

- 3/4 pound lean ground beef

- 1 minced onion

- 2 cloves garlic, crushed

- 10 ounces crushed tomatoes

For 3 pancakes:

- 3-4 tbsp skimmed milk

- 2-3 sparkle water

- salt

- 1 egg

- 1 and 2 tbsp cornstarch

For cheese layers:

- -18 ounces fat free cottage cheese (ricotta)

- 2 eggs

- 2 tbsp chopped fresh parsley

Directions:

1. Preheat oven to 375 degrees F (190 degrees C).

2. In a large skillet over medium heat brown the ground beef. Add the onion and garlic.
3. Stir in crushed tomatoes, tomato paste, tomato sauce, and water.
4. Season with basil, salt, pepper and the fresh parsley. Simmer, covered, for about 1 hour, stirring occasionally.

Butternut Squash & Carrot Puree

Ingredients:

- 1/8 teaspoon nutmeg

- Freshly ground black pepper, to taste

- 1 pound carrots, peeled and sliced into rounds

- 1 pound butternut squash, peeled and cubed

Directions:

1. Steam squash and carrots until tender, 5-7 minutes.
2. Transfer to blender or food processor and add nutmeg. Process until smooth.
3. Season with pepper to taste.

Tomato Oat Bran Gravy /Sauce

Ingredients:

- ½ tsp. paprika

- ½ tsp. cumin

- 2 Tbsp. fresh cilantro -chopped

- 1 clove garlic -purred

- 2 C roma tomatoes -chopped

- 1 ½ Tbsp. oat bran -grind into flour

- ½ - 2 C chicken stock

- ½ tsp. salt

Directions:

1. Toast oat flour in 300⬚ oven for 10 minutes stirring every 2 to 3 minutes, let it toast to desired color.
2. The darker it is toasted the nuttier it will taste.
3. Remove flour from oven and let cool. In a 2 qt stock pot add tomatoes and garlic, let come to a simmer.
4. In a bowl mix flour, salt, pepper, and chicken stock. Stir with a whisk to prevent lumps. Add the flour mixture to the tomatoes.
5. Set on medium heat and simmer until it thickens.
6. Use more or less liquid for a thicker or thinner sauce.

Yoghurt Cake

Ingredients:

- 4 tbsp oat bran

- 5 eggs

- 150g fat-free natural (or flavoured) yoghurt

- 6 tbsp powdered skimmed milk

- 2 tbsp Splenda granules

- 1 × 7g sachet dried yeast

- Flavouring of your choice

Directions:

1. Preheat the oven to 200C/Gas Mark 6 and line a 20cm (8in) loaf tin with greaseproof paper.

2. Process the oat bran as finely as possible using a blender or food processor and then combine with all the other Ingredients:.
3. Transfer the mixture to the tin.
4. Reduce the oven temperature to 180C/Gas Mark 4 and bake the cake for 35 minutes until lightly golden on top.

Red Pepper Fajitas And Chilli Chicken

Ingredients:

For the oat bran galette

- 1 teaspoon of dried thyme

- 1 finely chopped, green chilli pepper, seeds removed

- 2 whole eggs

- 4 tablespoons of 0% fat Greek yogurt

- 4 tablespoons of oat bran

For the chilli chicken

- 2 teaspoons of hot chilli powder

- 1 small onion

- 2 red peppers

- 2 small chicken breasts

- Low fat cream cheese

- A handful of chopped flat leaf parsley to serve

Directions:

1. Prepare the spicy oat bran galette, and add the thyme and chopped green chili to the batter before cooking. Set aside to cool when ready.
2. Chop the chicken into chunks, and slice the peppers and onion then mix all of them in a bowl.
3. Add in the chili powder while stirring to make sure that the peppers, chicken, and the onion are nicely flavored.
4. Preheat a griddle pan over high heat for about 5 minutes.

5. Place the chicken and vegetables on the griddle pan and cook until the meat turns golden brown.
6. Divide the oat bran galettes between two plates and uniformly spread with low fat cream cheese.
7. Top it with the spiced chicken, and add the chopped parsley to garnish. Serve when hot.

Chicken Supreme

Ingredients:

- 1 tbsp fat-free yogurt

- ½ tsp chives, chopped

- Salt, to taste

- Pepper, to taste

- ½ chicken breast, sliced

- ½ tsp Dijon mustard

- ½ glass of white wine

Directions:

1. In a pan, dry fry the sliced chicken pieces.
2. Add white wine to the pan and continue cooking, till the chicken is completely cooked.

3. Mix the mustard, yogurt, chives, salt and pepper in a separate bowl in order to achieve a sauce-like consistency.

4. Once the chicken has cooled, add the sauce to it.

Horseradish Dip

Ingredients:

- 5 teaspoon Horseradish

- ¼ teaspoon Pepper

- 1 teaspoon salt

- 250 grams Cauliflower

- 2 raw Eggs

Directions:

1. Cut the cauliflower into tiny pieces and put in a pot with 3/4 cup water.
2. Add salt, pepper and boil until the vegetable is soft. Remove pot from the heat.
3. Combine the cauliflower with one egg, mix and return to the range to cook for a while.
4. Throw in the second egg and blend again.

5. Put the horseradish and mix well and place it hot over the food you want to use it for.
6. Pour its leftover into a bottle to cool and use chilled with meals.

Cauliflower Pizzaiola

Ingredients:

- 200 g mozzarella

- Oregano, salt

- Extra virgin olive oil

- 1 cauliflower

- 150 ml tomato puree

Directions:

1. Take the cauliflower and wash it.
2. Remove the stem and leaves from the cauliflower and immerse it in lightly salted boiling water.
3. Cook the whole cauliflower for 5 minutes just to blanch it.
4. Drain the cauliflower and dry it well.

5. Cut the cauliflower into slices at least a finger thick and place them directly on a baking sheet with baking paper, drying them with paper towels.

6. Put the tomato puree on top of the cauliflower slices.

7. Drain the mozzarella from the water and crumble it with your hands.

8. Blot the mozzarella crumbs with paper towels to remove all the serum.

9. Place the mozzarella crumbs on top of the well-distributed cauliflower pizzas.

10. Dress the cauliflower pizzaiola with extra virgin olive oil, salt, and dried oregano.

11. Bake the cauliflower pizzaiola for 20 minutes in a preheated ventilated oven at 350° until the mozzarella has melted.

12. Remove the cauliflower pizzas from the oven and wait a couple of minutes before serving.

Coffee Frappuccino

Ingredients:

Oat bran:

- Egg whites, 2

- Spices of choice

- Oat bran, 3 tbsp

- Greek yogurt, 3 tbsp

Filling:

- Lean meat, cooked

- Cream cheese, low-fat, 2 tbsp

Directions:

1. In a bowl; add all Ingredients: together and whisk until form batter.
2. Add a bit of yogurt if batter is too thick; flavor with spices and favorite herbs.

3. Place half the mixture on frying pan coated with oil and cook until light brown.
4. Set aside.
5. Do the same for remaining mixture and arrange it on platters.
6. Halve galette and scatter cream on each sides.
7. Stuff cooked meat in there before you serve.

Chicken And Parsley Terrine

Ingredients:

- 1 large bunch of fresh parsley, stems removed, finely chopped

- 7 ounces cooked boneless, skinless chicken or turkey, diced

- 2 (7-gram) envelopes of unflavored gelatin

Directions:

1. In a small saucepan, mix the gelatin and 2 cups plus 1 tablespoon of cold water.
2. Bring the mixture to a boil slowly, stirring constantly.
3. As soon as the first bubbles appear, remove the pan from the heat and leave to cool.
4. Pour a thin layer of the gelatin into a loaf pan, cover, and put into the freezer for 3 minutes.

5. Combine the remaining gelatin mixture with the parsley and chicken.

6. Pour half of the chicken mixture into the loaf pan, cover, and freeze for 15 minutes.

7. Add the rest of the mixture to the loaf pan, cover, and refrigerate for 2 hours.

8. To turn the terrine out of the loaf pan, immerse the bottom of the pan into some hot water, then invert the loaf pan onto a large plate. The terrine will slide out.

Eggplant Parmesan

Ingredients:

- 1 medium eggplant (aubergine) you can peel them but i prefer mine with peel

Cooking spray

- 1 teaspoon dried oregano

- 1 teaspoon dried basil

- 2 egg white(s), lightly beaten

- 3 slices DD bread crumbed

- 1 Tbsp grated Parmesan cheese

- 1 teaspoon garlic powder

Sauce

- 1/2 teaspoon dried oregano

- 1/2 teaspoon dried basil

- 1 tablespoon tomato puree

- tin of chopped tomatoes

- 1/2 teaspoon garlic powder

- salt and pepper

- herbs of your choice for the sauce , i like italian seasoning in it

- 1/2 tspoon sweetener (it gives the sauce a more rounded flavour,)

- 1 diced onion,

- 1 very low fat laughing cow (optional)

Directions:

1. Preheat oven to 350°F. Spray a small baking dish with cooking spray; set aside.

87

2. Make up your tomato sauce, put tomatoes , herbs onions into a pan and cook until softened add tomato puree, 1/2 tsp sweetener and season to taste with salt and pepper, you will probably only need half the sauce for the dish but it keeps for several days in the fridge.

3. Combine bread crumbs, Parmesan cheese and herbs in a medium-size bowl; take a 1/4 of the mixture out to use as topping slice eggplant into 1/2-inch-thick slices.

4. Put them in a colander and sprinkle with salt, leave for 20 minutes, then rinse and pat dry with kitchen towels,

5. Dip eggplant first into egg whites and then into bread crumb mixture.

6. Bake eggplant on a nonstick baking sheet until lightly browned, about 20 to 25 minutes, flipping once.

7. Place a layer of eggplant on bottom of prepared baking dish, then add 1/3 of tomato sauce cheese.

8. Repeat until aubergine is all used , top with the last of the bread crumbs, dot with laughing cow cheese, Bake until cheese is melted and sauce is bubbling, about 10 minutes more.

Creamy Ham Egg Bake

Ingredients:

- 1 ½ c. fromage frais

- 6 cuts of ham, cleaved into little pieces

- Nutmeg, ocean salt and newly ground dark pepper

- ¾ c. skim milk

- 4 tsp. corn flour

- 4 eggs

Directions:

1. Preheat broiler to 450°F.
2. In an enormous bowl, consolidate milk and corn flour. Put away.

3. Then, separate egg whites from yolks. In a different bowl, beat egg yolks with fromage frais. Add yolks blend to milk and corn flour.
4. Mix until thick. Add ham, nutmeg, salt, and pepper to bowl. In another bowl, beat egg white until delicate pinnacles form.
5. Carefully overlay egg whites into yolk blend.
6. Heat for 45 minutes in a nonstick souffle or meal dish.

Kale Quinoa Salad

Ingredients:

- ½ avocado - peeled, pitted, and cut into cubes

- ½ tomato, cut into cubes

- ¼ cucumber, peeled and cut into cubes

- ¼ cup crumbled feta cheese

- 2 tablespoons Italian-style salad dressing

- ½ cup water

- ¼ cup quinoa

- 4 leaves kale, chopped, or more to taste

Directions:

1. Bring water and quinoa to a boil in a saucepan.

2. Reduce heat to medium-low, cover, and simmer until quinoa is tender, 15 to 20 minutes.
3. Drain water and run quinoa under cold water to cool.
4. Place a steamer insert into a saucepan and fill with water to just below the bottom of the steamer.
5. Bring water to a boil. Add kale, cover, and steam until tender, 2 to 3 minutes.
6. Place chopped kale in a bowl and refrigerate until chilled, 3 to 5 minutes.
7. Mix avocado, tomato, and cucumber together in a bowl; add quinoa and kale.
8. Sprinkle feta cheese over quinoa mixture; add Italian dressing and stir.

Divine Hard-Boiled Eggs

Ingredients:

- 12 eggs

Directions:

1. Place eggs in a pot; pour enough water over the eggs to cover.
2. Cover and turn stove to high; bring to a boil; turn off heat and place pot on a cool burner.
3. Let the pot sit with the cover on for 15 minutes.
4. Meanwhile, fill a large bowl halfway with cold water; transfer the eggs from the pot to the cold water.
5. Replace the water with cold water as needed to keep cold until the eggs are completely cooled.
6. Chill in refrigerator at least 2 hours before peeling.

Braised Tri-Tip

Ingredients:

- 1 cup beef broth

- 2 T dry minced onion, i love Penzey's

- 1 t Penzey's garlic powder

- 1 3 1/2 lb tri-tip

- 1/2 cup dry white wine

- 1/2 cup Worcestershire sauce

Directions:

1. Brown the meat in a large cast-iron pan with a bit of olive oil spray.

2. Place fat side down in the pan and season with the rest of the Ingredients:. Braise in an oven at 300 for 2-3 hours.

3. Slice and serve with pan juices. If you let the dish rest the sauce will be cool enough to strain.

4. Here's the trick: once the juices are cool, pour into a ziploc baggie. (do this over the sink) Once the fat has settled to the top, cut a tip of the corner of the baggie and let the good juices run into a measuring cup.

5. When you get close to the fat coming out, pull it away toward the sink.

6. Then you can reheat it all and you've skimmed most of the fat off!

Chicken And Tarragon Soup

Ingredients:

- 1 tablespoon dried skim milk

- 1 tablespoon cornflour (cornstarch) mixed with a little cold water

- Chicken stock cubes and 1 litre of water or 1 litre stock of your choice

- 1 large chicken breast or (any left over chicken)

- 1/2 diced onion

- 3 teaspoon dried tarragon,

Directions:

1. Cut up the chicken, into smallish pieces, add the onion and tarragon,bring it to the boil, turn down the heat and simmer until the

chicken is cooked and the onion is soft, about 15 mins

2. whiz it together with a hand blender until the chicken has broken up into smaller pieces or shreds, add the milk powder and cornflour, bring back to the boil, cook for 2 minutes to cook the cornflour, adjust seasoning to taste,

Dukan Crispy Stripes

Ingredients:

- 1 tbsp yogurt

- Salt, pepper, powdered garlic

- 2 tbsp oat bran

- 1 pound boneless, skinless chicken breast tenders

- 1 egg

Directions:

1. Preheat oven to 400 degrees F (200 degrees C). Lightly grease a 9×13 inch baking dish.
2. Cut the chicken breast into strips and sprinkle salt over them.
3. Beat the egg and mix it with the yogurt.
4. Add the salt, pepper and the garlic.
5. Dip chicken tenders in the mixture, then press in the oat bran to evenly coat.

6. Arrange in the prepared baking dish.

7. Bake 25 minutes in the preheated oven, or until chicken juices run clear.

Chicken And Vegetable Terrine

Ingredients:

- 1 yellow bell pepper, finely chopped

- 1-2 carrots, thinly sliced crosswise

- 1 cup of green bean

- 1 handful of bean yellow

- 500 g minced chicken (or turkey)

- 1 onion, finely chopped

- 1 egg, beaten

- Salt, pepper, paprika

Directions:

1. Preheat the oven to 180oC/350oF/Gas 4.

2. Steam the carrots, pepper and green bean for 5-6 minutes. In a large bowl combine chicken mince, egg, spring onions.

3. Add the steamed vegetables and stir.

4. Season the mixture to taste with salt and pepper.

5. Press the mixture firmly into a 22cm x 10cm baking paper lined loaf pan or a silicone tray.

6. Bake in a preheated oven for 45-50 minutes. Stand for 5 minutes before turning out of pan and slicing.

Hot Chocolate

Ingredients:

- 1 heaping tablespoon skim milk powder

- 8 oz skim milk

- 1 heaping teaspoon reduced fat, no sugar added cocoa powder

- Sweetener, to taste

Directions:

1. Place the cocoa powder and milk powder in a mug and mix well to combine.
2. Use a small amount of milk and mix into a paste.
3. Slowly stir in the rest of the milk, making sure that all Ingredients: are well-incorporated after each addition of milk.

4. Microwave for 1 minute on high and then add the sweetener.

5. Microwave for 1 minute more.

Eggnog

Ingredients:

- Vanilla extract, to taste

- Nutmeg & cinnamon, to taste

- 8 oz skim milk

- 1 egg yolk

- 2 teaspoons Splenda or other sweetener of
  your choice, to taste

Directions:

1. In microwaveable mug, heat milk on high for 1
   minute.
2. Meanwhile, in a small bowl, beat the
   sweetener and the egg yolk until creamy.
3. Very slowly, so as not to cook the egg yolk,
   stir the hot milk into the egg mixture a little at

a time, stirring constantly, until well-combined.

4. Add the vanilla extract and pour back into your mug.

5. If milk has cooled down too much, and you would like your eggnog warmer, microwave on medium for 30 seconds.

6. If you would like your eggnog chilled, cover your mug with transparent cling wrap and place it in the refrigerator for 30-60 minutes.

7. Top with a dusting of nutmeg and cinnamon prior to serving.

Chicken Tacos

Ingredients:

- ¼ tsp. kosher salt

- ¼ tsp. paprika

- 1 lb. boneless chicken -slice thin

- 1 tsp cumin

Directions:

1. Season chicken let marinate 30 minutes in refrigerator.
2. Place in nonstick baking dish. Bake on 400⬚ for 10 - 15 minutes. Let stand for 10 min.
3. Cut in thin strips and serve the chicken on romaine lettuce leaf, top with taco cabbage slaw (see recipe below) and cilantro.

Taco Cabbage Slaw

Ingredients:

- 2 Tbsp. tomato sauce

- 3 tsp. lime juice

- ½ tsp. kosher salt

- 2 c red cabbage -shredded

- 2 roma tomatoes

Directions:

1. Toss cabbage, tomatoes, lime juice and kosher salt.
2. Make ahead of time and let marinate to enhance the flavor.

Rotisserie Chicken & Sautéed Bok Choy

Ingredients:

- 2 Tbsp. chicken broth

- Salt & pepper to taste

- 2 - 4 C chicken -chopped, remove bones & skin

- 1 lb. Bok Choy -cut in quarters

Directions:

1. Use a nonstick skillet, add broth and Bok Choy sauté 2 to 3 minutes or until slightly wilted add chicken and heat.

2. Add salt and pepper to taste. Prep time 15 min; 2 servings

Chocolate And Mandarin Cereal Bars

Ingredients:

- 2 tsp mandarin flavouring

- 4 tsp sugar-free fat-reduced cocoa powder

- 1 tbsp fat-free fromage frais

- 8 tbsp oat bran

- 7 tbsp powdered skimmed milk

- 6 tbsp Canderel granules

- 3 tbsp water

Directions:

1. In a small bowl, combine the oat bran with 4 tbsp of the powdered skimmed milk, 3 tbsp of the Canderel, 2 tbsp of the water and the mandarin flavouring.

2. Mix everything together so that you get a smooth, compact paste.

3. Line a rectangular plastic container with clingfilm.

4. Spread the oat mixture evenly over the bottom and freeze for at least half an hour.

5. In another bowl, combine the cocoa powder with the remaining 3 tbsp powdered milk and 3 tbsp Canderel and the fromage frais. If necessary, add the remaining tbsp of water to get a semi-liquid cream.

6. Pour this cream over the oat bran and return to the freezer for at least 1 hour until it becomes hard.

7. Turn out of the container and cut into four bars. Store the bars in the fridge.

Italian-Style Strawberry Ice Cream

Ingredients:

- 40g virtually fat-free quark

- 2 tbsp low-fat single cream

- 1 tsp crystallised stevia

- 1 tsp strawberry flavouring (or any other flavouring of your choice)

- 3 eggs, separated

- Pinch salt

- 90g fat-free fromage frais

Directions:

1. In a bowl, beat the egg whites with the salt until stiff.

2. In a separate bowl, combine the egg yolks, fromage frais, quark, low-fat cream, stevia and strawberry flavouring.

3. Gently fold the beaten egg whites into the mixture.

4. Check that it is sufficiently sweet for your taste.

5. Transfer the mixture into two freezer-proof dishes and freeze for at least 2½ hours.

Nicoise Salad

Ingredients:

- 2 hard-boiled eggs

- A handful of green beans, fresh or frozen

- 1/2 butternut squash (optional)

- A drizzle of balsamic vinegar

- 2 small salad tomatoes, sliced

- 1 bag of mixed leaves salad

- 1 large can of tuna in brine (185g)

Directions:

1. Pre-heat the oven to 180 degrees C.

2. Skin, then cut the butternut squash into smaller cubes and place on a baking tray lined with greaseproof paper.

114

3. Spray with low fat cooking spray and cook in the pre-heated oven for some 40 minutes until tender.

4. Put the green beans in a food steamer and cook as per the manufacturer's instructions.

5. Steaming is highly recommended to ensure that there is minimal loss of vitamins and nutrients. You can also cook in the microwave or boil them in hot water until soft.

6. Hard-boil the eggs in boiling water for about 10 minutes while you wait for the green beans to cook.

7. Start preparing the salad when the eggs are set and the green beans have cooled down.

8. First, place the salad on a plate then add the tomatoes, the butternut squash and the green beans.

9. Divide the eggs into quarter bits, and top them on salad.

10. Place the drained tuna on top then spread with balsamic vinegar.

Tomato Eggs

Ingredients:

- 400g can of chopped tomatoes

- Salt and pepper

- A few roughly chopped leaves of fresh basil

- 4 eggs

- Vegetable oil spray

- Half a large onion, chopped

- 3 tablespoons of warm water

Directions:

1. Spray a non-stick pan with vegetable oil spray then heat it over medium heat and gently fry the onions until translucent.

2. Add 3 tablespoons of water and tomatoes, and mix well. Let these cook while covered on low heat for 10-15 minutes.
3. Add a little more water if the sauce starts to get too thick and sticky.
4. Add the basil and stir well to make sure that tomatoes absorb the sweet basil aroma.
5. Break the eggs and pour at the top of the sauce then add salt and pepper to taste and cover again.
6. You will know if the eggs are ready when the egg whites turn solid while the yolk is still runny.

Baked Egg Custard

Ingredients:

- 2 tbsp sweetener

- 1 tsp almond extract

- ½ tbsp vanilla essence

- Pinch of salt

- 3 eggs

- 2 egg whites

- 3 cups skimmed milk

Directions:

1. Preheat oven at 275 °F.
2. Boil the milk – keep stirring so it does not stick to the bottom of the container.

3. Stir sweetener and salt, till they totally dissolve.

4. In a bowl, beat the eggs. Then add almond extract and vanilla essence. Add the hot milk while still beating the mixture.

5. Pour equal quantities of this mixture into ramekins. Place them in a pan – and pour boiling water till half the height of the ramekin.

6. Bake for about an hour, till the custards become firm in the edges.

7. Let it cool; then refrigerate.

Steak Au Poivre

Ingredients:

- 2 tbsp skimmed milk

- 4 tbsp zero-fat fromage frais

- ½ tbsp Dijon mustard

- 2 beef tenderloin steaks

- 1 tbsp black peppercorns, crushed

- ½ onion, finely chopped

- Salt, to taste

Directions:

1. Season the steaks with salt, and let it stand for half an hour.
2. Then, coat the steaks with black peppercorns.

3. In a pan, dry fry the steaks, till it is cooked to your liking.

4. Wrap the steaks with foil and set aside.

5. Next, fry the onion in a pan till it becomes soft. Simultaneously, in another pan, heat milk and add Dijon mustard to it.

6. Remove this from the heat and add milk and fromage frais. When they have combined completely, continue heating it.

7. Place the steak on plates, and pour this sauce over it.

Kale Blueberry Smoothie

Ingredients:

- 1/2 cup Ice

- A cup of kale

- ½ cup nonfat vanilla Greek yogurt

- A tablespoon of almond butter

- 1 cup frozen blueberries

Directions:

1. Mix all in a blender and blend till smooth.

Oat Fiber Zucchini Muffins

Ingredients:

- 1.5 cups Oat bran

- 1 tablespoon pumpkin spice

- 1 cup Splenda

- 1 tablespoon Vanilla extract

- 1 cup fresh, grated and with juice Zucchini

- 1 teaspoon Baking soda

- 1 tablespoon low fat, unsweetened cocoa powder

- ½ cup nonfat Milk

- 1/3 cup nonfat Greek yogurt

- 3 Large Eggs

Directions:

1. Place oven to 350◦C. Mix wet and arid Ingredients: in two separate containers.

2. Put dry to wet slowly while combining with a spoon.

3. Streak a large muffin sheet with paper cups and put mixture into every cup evenly.

4. Cook for 20 minutes. This recipe makes a dozen muffins.

Bresaola And Rocket Baskets

Ingredients:

- 150 g ricotta cheese

- 60 g parmesan cheese, 10 g rocket To decorate: rocket balsamic vinegar glaze

- 1 puff pastry roll, 100 g Bresaola

Directions:

1. Unroll the puff pastry and roll it out on a work surface.
2. Cut circles with a pastry cutter or a pastry cup and place them in lightly oiled muffin molds.
3. Punch holes in the base of the baskets so that they don't puff up during baking.
4. Place a piece of parchment paper over the puff pastry disks and place a weight on top.
5. Bake the puff pastry baskets in a preheated ventilated oven for 10 minutes at 180

degrees, then remove the parchment paper and cook for about 5 minutes more until golden brown.

6. Remove the puff pastry baskets from the oven and let them cool completely.

7. Place the ricotta and Parmesan in a bowl and mix.

8. Chop the arugula and add it to the ricotta in the bowl, stirring with a spoon.

9. Take the cooled puff pastry baskets and place a slice of Bresaola then add a few leaves of arugula and place a ball of ricotta and arugula in the center.

10. Decorate with balsamic vinegar glaze.

Pancakes Potatoes And Leeks

Ingredients:

- 2 leeks, salt

- 70 g parmesan cheese

- 1 egg, flour 00

- 400 g potatoes

- Extra virgin olive oil

- Peanut seed oil

Directions:

1. Wash the potatoes with the peel and put them in a pot of cold water.

2. Put the pot on the stove and cook the potatoes until they are cooked and soft. Mash the potatoes while still hot with a potato masher and place them in a bowl.

3. Cut the ends off the leeks and slice them into small pieces.

4. Heat two tablespoons of extra virgin olive oil in a skillet and cook the leeks.

5. Season lightly with salt and cook the leeks for about 10 minutes, then turn off the heat and add the cooked leeks to the mashed potatoes.

Homemade Yogurt

Ingredients:

- Jelly, sugar-free, 3 tsp

- Boiling water, 3 tsp

- Yogurt, fat-free, 1 large tub

Directions:

1. Take a bowl; add boiling water and whisk jelly properly until properly dissolved.

2. Keep it aside for about 3 minutes and to chill.

3. In a food processor; add jelly syrup as well as yogurt and process until smooth before you serve.

Keto Sweet Broccoli Salad

Ingredients:

- ¼ cup chopped green onions

- 3 tablespoons sunflower seeds

- ½ cup mayonnaise

- ¼ cup low-calorie natural sweetener (such as Swerve®)

- 3 tablespoons apple cider vinegar

- 5 slices bacon

- 1 head broccoli, cut into bite-size pieces

- ½ cup grated sharp Cheddar cheese

Directions:

1. Place bacon in a large skillet and cook over medium-high heat, turning occasionally, until evenly browned, about 10 minutes.

2. Drain bacon slices on paper towels. Crumble once cool enough to handle.

3. Combine bacon, broccoli, Cheddar cheese, green onions, and sunflower seeds in a large bowl.

4. Stir mayonnaise, sweetener, and apple cider vinegar together in a small bowl.

5. Pour dressing over broccoli mixture and toss until well combined.

Air Fryer Gluten-Free Fried Chicken

Ingredients:

- 1 ¼ cups gluten free crackers

- 2 pounds boneless, skinless chicken breast, cut in 1-inch pieces

- ¼ cup vegetable oil

- 6 large eggs

- Salt and freshly ground black pepper to taste

- 1 ¼ cups gluten-free flour

Directions:

1. Whisk eggs in a shallow bowl and season with salt and pepper.
2. Place flour in a second bowl and cracker crumbs in a third bowl.

3. Dredge chicken pieces first in flour, then in eggs, and finally in cracker crumbs.

4. Place on an air fryer rack, making sure pieces don't touch. Brush tops of chicken with oil.

5. Air fry chicken at 375 degrees F (190 degrees C) until cooked through and crisp, about 10 minutes.

Easy Grilled Chicken Wings

Ingredients:

- 3 teaspoons garlic salt

- 3 teaspoons ground black pepper

- 20 chicken wings

- 2 tablespoons olive oil, or more as needed

Directions:

1. Preheat an outdoor grill for high heat and lightly oil the grate

2. Tuck in the chicken wing flaps so the wing forms a triangle.

3. Combine olive oil with some of the garlic salt and pepper in a large bowl.

4. Add a few chicken wings and turn to coat with seasonings.

5. Add more wings, remaining garlic salt, and remaining pepper and turn to coat. Repeat until all wings are coated. Place on the preheated grill.

6. Grill until wings are well browned, tender, and no longer pink at the bone and juices run clear, turning several times and rearranging them so they cook evenly, 30 to 40 minutes.

Crepes

Ingredients:

- ⅔ cup all-purpose flour

- 1 pinch salt

- 1 ½ teaspoons vegetable oil

- 2 eggs

- 1 cup milk

Directions:

1. In a blender combine eggs, milk, flour, salt and oil.
2. Process until smooth. Cover and refrigerate 1 hour.
3. Heat a skillet over medium-high heat and brush with oil.
4. Pour 1/4 cup of crepe batter into pan, tilting to completely coat the surface of the pan.

5. Cook 2 to 5 minutes, turning once, until golden. Repeat with remaining batter.

White Sauce

Ingredients:

- 1 small pot non-fat yoghurt

- Salt and pepper

- 125ml (4fl oz) skimmed milk

- 2 egg yolks, beaten

Directions:

1. In a double saucepan, heat the milk until lukewarm the add salt and pepper. Pour a small amount of the milk over the egg yolks, then incorporate the eggs and milk mixture into the pan.

2. Beat well and add the yoghurt. Heat the sauce through.

3. If serving with fish you can add some chopped gherkin.

Creamy Currry Sauce

Ingredients:

- 10 grams mustard of choice

- 1 tea spoon curry powder of choice

- 80 grams fat free fromage frais

Directions:

1. Mixed all Ingredients: together.
2. Can be served straight away, or put in microwave for 30-60 second to take off chill.

Chicken Meatballs

Ingredients:

- Spices (salt, pepper, garlic powder)

- 2 tbsp oat bran

- 3 tablespoons finely chopped flat-leaf parsley or dill

- 1 pound ground chicken

- 1 small onion, finely chopped

- 1 small garlic clove, minced

- 1 large egg

Directions:

1. Preheat the oven to 180oC/350oF/Gas 4.

2. Mince your onion and garlic or put them in a food processor if you don't want to chop them.
3. Add all the ingredients in a large bowl and mix together (you can also mix by hand).
4. Form mixture into 15-20 meatballs; place on prepared pan.
5. Bake in centre of preheated oven until juices run clear, 18 to 20 minutes.
6. On your PV days you can eat it with peperonata.

Chicken Meatballs

Ingredients:

- 1 large egg

- Spices (salt, pepper, garlic powder)

- 2 tbsp oat bran

- 3 tablespoons finely chopped flat-leaf parsley or dill

- 1 pound ground chicken

- 1 small onion, finely chopped

- 1 small garlic clove, minced

Directions:

1. Preheat the oven to 180oC/350oF/Gas 4.

2. Mince your onion and garlic or put them in a food processor if you don't want to chop them.

3. Add all the Ingredients: in a large bowl and mix together (you can also mix by hand).

4. Form mixture into 15-20 meatballs; place on prepared pan.

5. Bake in centre of preheated oven until juices run clear, 18 to 20 minutes. On your PV days you can eat it with peperonata.

6. Enjoy my dukan recipe!

Floating Islands

Ingredients:

- Vanilla extract, to taste

- Sweetener, to taste

- Nutmeg, to taste

- 4 separated eggs

- 18 oz skim milk

Directions:

1. Starting with room temperature eggs, beat the egg whites in a small bowl until you get soft, but firm peaks that stay standing when you lift your beater.

2. Put the milk, sweetener and vanilla extract into a saucepan and slowly bring to a boil over low heat. You want to do this slowly so that you don't scald the milk.

145

3. Carefully spoon out snowball-sized portions of the egg whites and float them in the hot milk mix, where they will become poached.

4. Turn the egg white balls one time, let them cook for a few minutes, and then remove them with a slotted spoon to drain on a plate.

5. Beat the egg yolks in a medium bowl and – slowly – add the milk mixture to the bowl a little at a time to avoid cooking the eggs, stirring constantly.

6. Return the milk/egg mixture to the saucepan and keep stirring, over low heat, until it starts to set up and the custard is formed.

7. To serve, you can pour some custard into individual bowls and top each with an egg white "floating island" or you can leave all the custard in one big bowl with many floating islands on top.

Tomato & Basil Relish

Ingredients:

- ¼ C basil -fresh, chopped

- ½ tsp. balsamic vinegar

- Salt & black pepper

- 1 C plum tomatoes -diced

- 2 Tbsp. red onion -diced

- ¼ C pimientos -drain, diced

Directions:

1. Mix tomatoes, onions, pimientos, and basil together in a small bowl.

Zucchini And Feta Appetizer

Ingredients:

- 2 eggs

- ½ block of low-fat feta cheese (tolerated)

- ½ bunch of basil

- Sea salt, black pepper

- 3 tablespoons Dukan Diet Oat Bran

- 1 zucchini

- 1 onion

Directions:

1. Preheat the oven to 425°F. Grate the zucchini without peeling it.

2. Thinly slice the onion, chop up the basil very finely and crumble the feta. In a large bowl,

combine the zucchini, onion, basil, feta cheese, oat bran, eggs and add salt and black pepper.

3. Once the mixture is well blended, spoon out small balls onto a baking sheet covered with parchment paper.

4. Bake for 15 minutes then remove from the oven, turn the appetizers over and bake for a further 15 minutes

Dukan Cocktail

Ingredients:

- 1 tablespoon of chopped chives

- A pinch of paprika

- 1 tablespoon of Tabasco sauce (optional)

- A squeeze of lemon juice

- 200g of 0% fat Greek yogurt

- 150g of cooked cocktail prawns

Directions:

1. Pour the Greek yogurt in a bowl and blend in the chopped chives, lemon juice, Tabasco sauce and paprika.

2. Mix well until all ingredients have blended, and then blend in the prawns until they are fully covered with the sauce.

3. Sprinkle with paprika and serve when cold.

CPSIA information can be obtained
at www.ICGtesting.com
Printed in the USA
LVHW080914171222
735289LV00010BA/2227